MW00618865

with ~ *Jelle*

9/18

Early
arrival

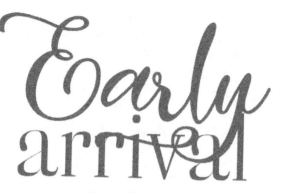

Early arrival

9 Things Parents Need to Know
about Life in the ICU Nursery:

A Doctor's Step-by-Step Guide

TERRI MAJOR-KINCADE, MD, MPH

purposely
created
PUBLISHING

EARLY ARRIVAL

Published by Purposely Created Publishing Group™

Copyright © 2018 Terri Major-Kincade

Printed in the United States of America
ISBN: 978-1-948400-55-8

DEDICATION

This book is dedicated to the hundreds of babies and families that I have had the pleasure of caring for over the past twenty years. There is nothing quite like holding a tiny human in your hand and watching that tiny human one day grow big enough and strong enough to go home with their parents... who are in fact the strongest of all. If you are holding this book, I imagine you or someone near to you has found themselves down the rabbit hole... in the tunnel... on the roller coaster known as the NICU, or Neonatal Intensive Care Unit. Take a deep breath. Exhale. I am here to hold your hand... one step at a time, one day at a time. There will be good days and, sadly, some bad days too, but you are not alone.

A special dedication to my baby sister, the first preemie I ever loved and my inspiration for becoming a neonatologist. It's a blessing I don't take for granted... thank you for letting me be part of your journey.

TABLE OF CONTENTS

INTRODUCTION

This book has been in my heart for many years. It carries with it the face and soul of every parent whose eyes I have ever looked into and said: "Hi, I'm Dr. Terri. Your obstetrician asked me to speak with you... about the possible delivery of your preterm baby. I'm here to talk to you about what to expect if we meet your baby today. Hopefully, your baby will be able to stay in just a little bit longer, but if not I will be here to help you and your baby."

My sister was born three months early in 1968, only a couple of years after President Kennedy lost his son to prematurity. I've often wondered who spoke with my parents. Did they understand the magnitude of what it meant to have a one-pound baby, three months early? Can anyone, other than those going through it or those who have experienced it, understand the magnitude of those moments when emotions are high, belief is suspended, and time is passing by? I think not. My sister's early arrival is what motivated and inspired me to want to become a preemie doctor, a neonatologist. I was fascinated by the fact that, when she was born, she could fit into the palm of your hand and that she slept in a plastic box called an incubator. I wanted to take care of those babies and help those families.

I've achieved my dream, but my achieving my dream means that every day I will meet someone who wasn't planning to meet me. Who doesn't want to meet me… because to meet me means that you are having a baby that may be very sick. My job is not just caring for babies, but caring for their families too. I wrote this book as a way to help care for families who hear the words: "You're having a premature baby." In *Early Arrival* you will learn about the world of the neonatal intensive care unit, the people who work in the intensive nursery, the equipment used to care for your baby, the most common problems of premature babies, and how to prepare to take your baby home. Sometimes, sadly, babies do not get to go home… so yes, I will hold your hand through that as well. I hope and pray with all of my heart that you find this book helpful and that your Early Arrival will bless your family. All the best on your journey.

Sincerely, Dr. Terri, MD

CHAPTER 1

Who Is Caring for My Baby?

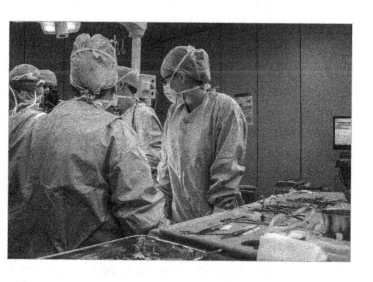

Welcome to the neonatal intensive care unit, or NICU as it's more commonly known. It's a land of bells, whistles, alarms, machines, and many, many people charged with caring for tiny, tiny humans, and it can all be quite over-whelming until you get used to it. Some parents would say that you never really get used to it... but you learn to navigate your way through the sounds, through the wires, through the machines, and, yes, through the peo-ple to finally connect with your baby... as you should. After all, you are the parents—you are, in fact, Mom and Dad—but so many people are making so many decisions each day that sometimes it's hard to figure out where you might fit in. But trust me, you do fit in, and learning the cast of players will hopefully help you to find your place more quickly. We are waiting for you... and so is your baby. Parents are definitely part of the health care team, don't ever forget that... and, if needed, remind your health care partners every now and then! It really makes a difference.

So who are the members of the health care team that are charged with caring for your infant in the NICU? This may vary, depending upon whether your baby is in a Level III or Level IV ICU nursery—ones that care for the sickest and smallest of infants, usually those born at less than twenty-eight weeks or three pounds, who may ultimately require surgery and access to subspecialists—or in a Level II NICU that cares for bigger preemies, usu-ally those born at greater than thirty-two weeks or larger than three pounds, who require more minimal support. But, for the most part, some general categories can be found with respect to caregivers in the NICU.

The physician charged with caring for babies in the NICU is called a neonatologist. A **neonatologist** is a physician who has trained in pediatrics as well as completed an additional three years of training in neo-natal-perinatal medicine. They specialize in the care of both sick term infants and sick preterm infants. A term pregnancy is defined as a pregnancy that is thirty-seven weeks or more. Most people think of pregnancy as last-ing nine months, but a full-term pregnancy is actually forty weeks. Any infant born at less than thirty-seven weeks is considered to be preterm. This is important be-cause, although most people think of the one- and two-pound babies when they think of preterm infants, the majority of babies in neonatal intensive care units are the bigger preemies… especially those preemies between thirty-four and thirty-six weeks, who are referred to as late preterm.

Neonatologists often work very closely with **neona-tal nurse practitioners**. Neonatal nurse practitioners, or NNPs, are neonatal nurses who have specialized train-ing in the care of sick preterm or term infants and, in some instances, are authorized to act independently in the care and stabilization of neonates.

Respiratory therapists are therapists who specialize in the stabilization and support of your baby's lungs through the setup and maintenance of key equipment and therapies. Some of this equipment includes a respirator or ventilator to breathe for your baby and a nasal cannula or nasal CPAP to provide oxygen therapy. A respirator or ventilator is a machine that is used to actually breathe for the baby if the baby is too small or too sick to breathe on his or her own. If the baby is not as sick, a nasal CPAP may be used. CPAP stands for continuous positive airway pressure. Many adults are familiar with CPAP, as a similar machine is prescribed for home use in adults who may have obstructive sleep apnea. In premature babies who are able to breathe on their own but may require a little additional help to keep their lungs open, a nasal CPAP may be used instead of a respirator. Additionally, many premature infants will require breathing treatments for wheezing, chest physical therapy for secretions, or suctioning, all of which are provided by the respiratory therapist.

The **bedside neonatal nurse** is the caregiver that parents will become the most familiar with and, perhaps, the most bonded to. The bedside nurse will be caring for your infant for up to twelve hours a day and will become very familiar with your infant's baseline, as well as with you as parents. In many ways, they become like family. In addition to caring for the infant's basic medical needs, watching vital signs, feeding the infant, making sure the infant is comfortable, and providing emotional support to families, the neonatal nurse plays a key role in identifying sudden changes in the infant that may require emergency intervention.

Lactation support is generally a nurse whose primary role is to support and encourage breast milk production for the mother and to support direct breastfeeding once an infant is stable enough to directly breastfeed. Breast milk is considered to be vital to the development and growth of all babies, but it is particularly important for premature babies in the prevention of significant and life-threatening infections. Most preemies are not able to latch on for some time, but lactation support can help a mother to ensure that her milk supply is well established so that an infant can receive milk through a feeding tube until he or she is ready to breastfeed.

Neonatal physical and occupational therapists are essential to the normal development of preterm infants and term infants in the NICU. However, most of their duties happen later in the NICU stay, once the infant is in less critical condition. A big role for the occupational therapist is helping the infant to feed without choking. Most infants know how to suck and swallow, but to suck, swallow, and breathe without choking is a function of maturity. Infants and parents often require support to learn the technique of feeding premature infants carefully to avoid choking. Premature babies develop their suck reflex very early, and can even be seen sucking in the womb as early as twenty-four weeks. However, to suck and swallow without choking is a skill that develops over time, and often does not mature until thirty-six to thirty-eight weeks. The occupational therapist is instrumental in teaching families to watch how the baby sucks, breathes, and swallows, as well as to slow the baby down when he or she is doing more sucking than breathing or continuing to suck without swallowing. This is known as pacing. Additionally, a physical therapist might be needed to develop range-of-motion exercises and other techniques for infants that might have sustained a brain injury or for whom there may be a later concern for developmental challenges.

Another key member of the medical team in the NICU is the **social worker**. Often the social worker is one of the first people that you meet once your child is admitted to the NICU. He or she will be able to provide you with valuable resources for parents in the NICU, as well as referrals if additional help is required, such as identifying solutions to transportation or housing barriers during the NICU stay. Also, if an infant being discharged requires equipment such as oxygen assistance, as many preemies do, the social worker will have helped with setting up the training to use the equipment and with expediting the discharge process.

Finally, the last and most important member of the health care team is YOU. It may not seem like it... but you are. You are the parent advocate. You will be presented with information and asked to weigh in on different treatment options. You will get to know each of the other members of the health care team and hopefully build trust during your NICU stay, which will allow you to more comfortably and confidently weigh in on treatment decisions that affect the overall progress of your child. It's normal to be afraid. It's normal to be overwhelmed... but I know you can do it, and your baby's team is here to support you through that. So go for it... get to know the team. We are ready to meet you!

Questions for My Baby's Doctor

_____

_____

_____

_____

_____

_____

_____

Notes about My Baby

_____

_____

_____

_____

_____

_____

_____

CHAPTER 2

One Baby, Many Tubes

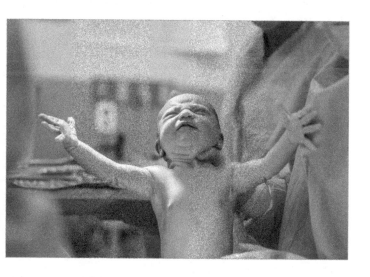

One of the biggest challenges for parents when first entering the NICU is getting used to seeing their sick baby connected to so many tubes and wires. It can be quite humbling to see a baby fighting to breathe... tiny ribs going in and out, tiny hands and feet moving, grasping, fighting, and a tiny voice or cry often unheard because the breathing tube is in place. Often, it's hard to actually see the baby because of the machines, or even to process what the physician, nurse practitioner, or nurse may be saying because of the noise. But after a time, you will become more comfortable with the noise and, yes, the machines too. One day you will hopefully walk into the NICU and see one less machine connected to your baby. You will see one less wire and hear one less alarm. Cherish those moments, because they mean that your baby is one step closer to going home.

But in the meantime, what do the machines mean? What are the wires? Which pieces of equipment are you most likely to see connected to your baby? Some of the equipment that will be used to help stabilize your infant will, of course, be related to the specific diagnosis. But many of the items that are used to help babies in the NICU are standard for all babies, and those are the items we will emphasize in this chapter.

One of the most common items is a **breathing tube**. Many premature and term infants may require help breathing. A special tube can be placed to breathe for the baby; it goes through the baby's mouth, down the baby's throat, and through the windpipe, staying just past the vocal cords and Adam's apple at the trachea, which connects to both bronchi and leads to the lungs. If the breathing tube is in the right place, you will not be able to hear the baby cry, because it passes between the vocal cords and keeps them open. After the breathing tube is placed, it will be connected to a **respirator** or **ventilator** machine, which will help the baby to breathe until the baby is more stable. There are many types of breathing machines. Your physician and nurse practitioner will determine which machine is best for your baby.

Some babies can breathe on their own but still need a little help, either because of immaturity or because they may have fluid in their lungs, and need a little oxygen. For those babies, something called a **nasal cannula**, which is a small plastic tubing, may be placed on their face over their nose to provide oxygen and to stimulate the baby to breathe. Some babies may require additional help and can be placed on a **nasal CPAP**, which looks like either two small plastic prongs that can be placed in the baby's nose or a small plastic mask that can be placed over the baby's nose. As mentioned earlier, CPAP stands for continuous positive airway pressure. Many parents are already familiar with CPAP because they may know an adult who sleeps on a CPAP machine at night for sleep apnea.

A **temperature sensor**, often shaped like a gold duck or a gold heart, will be attached to the baby's abdomen. It will signal to the incubator or warmer if the baby is too cold or too hot and allow the machine to adjust itself accordingly to keep your baby comfortable.

A **feeding tube** may be placed through the baby's nose or mouth to help keep air out of the tummy and to provide the baby with food into the stomach. This is necessary either if the baby is not old enough to breast-feed or take a bottle or if the baby is too unstable to feed by mouth.

Many sick babies will initially require intravenous (IV) fluids because they will be too sick to eat and will require fluids to keep them stable until they are ready to eat. In bigger babies, they may have a regular IV very similar to the one that the mother had, known as a **peripheral IV**. If the baby is small or more unstable, he or she may require a more invasive line, known as a central line, which will pass deeper than just the skin. This line may be placed through the umbilical cord, through the groin, through the lower leg, through the arm, or into the neck. It is called a central line because it starts outside the body and ends up in a central location in the chest. Most premature babies will begin with an **umbilical intravenous line** and then change to a different central line called a **PICC** (peripherally inserted central catheter) once they are older. They will continue to have these lines until they are stable or are able to receive full nutrition from formula or breast milk.

Most premature and term babies will begin on a **radiant warmer**, which looks like an open type bed that allows the doctors and nurses to be able to reach the baby quickly. Once the baby is more stable, the baby will be in an **isolette** or **incubator** if he or she is too small for a regular crib. The isolette or incubator looks like a small plastic box with portholes that allow you to see and to touch your baby without the baby getting too cold.

At some point, you are sure to notice a **special blue light** on either your baby or one of the many other babies in the NICU. All babies have jaundice (also called hyperbilirubinemia), which may or may not be visible. Jaundice is the term doctors or nurses may use to refer to the skin of your baby, which may appear redder or more yellow. The jaundice color is related to the products from the breakdown of old blood, known as bilirubin. When the blood is broken down, it is cleared through the liver. This process in a full-term baby who is well usually occurs over three to seven days. In a premature baby, this process may take longer because they are not eating as much and therefore are not having as many bowel movements. Additionally, preemies may be more dehydrated due to their thinner skin, which can also cause the process to take longer. There are other causes of hyperbilirubinemia as well that may result in a longer-than-expected period of jaundice. If this is the case, your health care team will discuss other options for treatment. For routine (or physiologic) jaundice, the liver is the primary way the body removes the bilirubin. To do its job well, the liver needs adequate fluid, which can be a problem if the baby is unable to eat, and it takes most preemies and sick babies a while for the liver to figure out how to do this. For most babies, sick and healthy, jaundice is a normal physiological occurrence. In some babies, if the jaundice or bilirubin number is higher than we would anticipate, we can place the baby under a special blue light (**phototherapy light**) that uses UV light to break the bilirubin down in the skin and allow the baby to get rid of the bilirubin.

Lastly, what about the alarms? There must be about a million each day, right? Well, that might be a bit of an exaggeration, but there are quite a few. Those of us who work in the NICU daily become used to them, and we are quite used to caring for and responding to your baby when the need arises. I want to assure you that if you are in the NICU and you hear alarms going off, we are paying attention, even if seems like we are not! There are two primary alarms in the NICU. One is the alarm for the **cardiorespiratory monitor**. It will signal whenever the baby has an extended period of a low or elevated heart rate or an extended period of no respirations, also known as apnea. The second most common alarm is the alarm that is attached to the **pulse oximetry machine**. It is the red bulb usually attached to the baby's foot or hand in a blue Velcro wrap. It will let the medical team know how well your baby is using the oxygen, also known as how saturated the blood is with oxygen. This alarm goes off frequently, as it is designed to monitor a steady pulse signal, and often, if the baby is kicking or moving, the signal may be momentarily disrupted. The pulse oximetry alarm is not a perfect machine and works best if a baby is perfectly still or sleeping. It is not uncommon for the alarm to go off if the baby is kicking or crying, as it is trying to find a steady pulse or signal from the baby. Often, the baby has settled down after a few seconds and the signal is reestablished. In those instances, you may notice that your nurse or provider may only casually glance at the alarm or the baby but not necessarily intervene. Not every alarm requires intervention. Your health care team is very familiar with the alarms, and it will take a while for you to get used to them. If you do not see an immediate response to an alarm for your infant, it does not mean that no one is paying attention. The nurses and the providers will get to know your baby very well… and so will you. Eventually, you will be accustomed to the alarms that will be routine for your baby, and as your baby grows older, we can expect to hear and see fewer and fewer alarms.

Questions for My Baby's Doctor

_____

_____

_____

_____

_____

_____

Notes about My Baby

_____

_____

_____

_____

_____

_____

CHAPTER 3

About the
Preemie Lungs

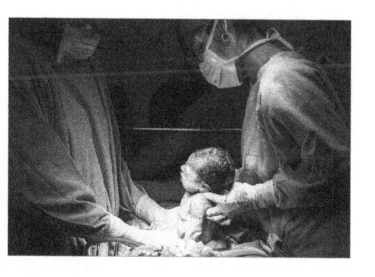

Having a baby that is admitted to the NICU is very scary, whether the baby is premature, very small, and expected to be sick, or whether the baby is term but has to be transferred to the intensive care nursery emergently. A premature baby is often expected to have problems with breathing that will require admission to the ICU nursery. A baby that is full term is not normally expected to be admitted to the ICU nursery. Sometimes, though, things can happen right at the time of delivery that will cause the infant to have trouble breathing, including breech presentation, the umbilical cord around the neck, bleeding in the mother, or fluid in the baby's lungs. Any of these conditions can cause a term baby to be suddenly admitted to the NICU.

There are many, many reasons why a baby may have to be admitted to the NICU, but before any condition can be assessed the medical team will need to stabilize the baby. In the delivery room, the main focus will be on the baby's heart rate and the baby's breathing. If we are unable to help the baby to breathe, the heart rate will not stabilize. If the heart rate does not stabilize, the baby will not survive. So, breathing is number one on the list for the medical team. We want your baby to breathe. We want your baby to cry. And hopefully, if your baby can breathe, if your baby can cry, the heart rate will stabilize. If we can stabilize those two systems, it will give us time to determine what other support your baby will require. It can be scary to know that your baby needs helps with breathing.

It can also be disheartening to see your baby on a breathing machine. But breathing problems are one of the most common problems to be managed in the intensive care unit nursery, and your team will know best when it is time to remove the breathing support from your baby. Until then, try to hang in there, Mom and Dad. Inhale, exhale, breathe… one day, one shift at a time.

Most premature babies, even the tiny ones, if delivered stable, will have some respiratory effort, will be able to breathe. But often they get tired after the initial cry and the initial attempts to expand their lungs. The lungs in a preterm baby are initially very stiff, and this stiffness typically does not improve until after the baby has been developing for thirty-seven weeks. We can give mothers medicine to improve this, such as steroids, and we can also give babies a special protein to improve this, such as surfactant, but premature babies and some term babies can still have many challenges with breathing which must be evaluated on a daily basis. If the baby becomes tired from breathing when in the delivery room or in the NICU, we are, in most cases, able to offer the baby additional help. This help includes oxygen therapy via a nasal cannula or nasal CPAP and the use of a respirator or ventilator. Both premature babies and term babies may require this type of support.

The most common problems with breathing for premature babies include respiratory distress syndrome; pneumonia; retained fetal lung fluid (all babies will have fluid in their lungs, but some babies have a harder time clearing the fluid); meconium aspiration (if the baby had a bowel movement prior to delivery); and lung collapse. Additionally, babies may have other complications related to genetics or chromosomes that may require special testing.

Questions for My Baby's Doctor

Notes about My Baby

CHAPTER 4

Infection, Infection, Infection

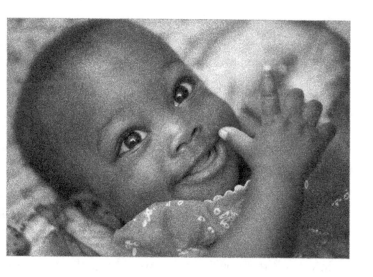

When babies are admitted to the intensive care nursery, the most common question parents understandably ask is, "Is my baby going to be okay?" In that moment, what most parents really want to know is, "Will my baby survive? Will I be able to take my baby home?" Fortunately, most bigger preemies and most term infants that are admitted to the neonatal intensive care unit have conditions that respond favorably to treatment. Unfortunately, not all babies respond, and occasionally babies are born with conditions for which there is no treatment. But in the moment that parents ask those very loaded questions, most of our responses operate under the assumption that we will be able to stabilize your baby. That we will be able to help your baby breathe. That the major organ systems, especially the heart and lungs, will respond to either management or medications targeted for your baby's specific condition. However, even in the best case scenario, and even with attempts to treat them in the intensive care nursery, many of the babies who do not survive will die due to infection.

Having a baby who has a severe viral or bacterial infection is a true medical emergency, and for a premature baby, the stakes are even higher. Babies do not have a fully developed immune system, so they are more prone to infections from bacteria that would not affect healthy adults. Additionally, in babies the barriers between body cavities are not as established, and it is very easy for bacteria to infect the lungs, the urinary tract, the bloodstream, or the intestines and go on to affect the spinal cord and, ultimately, cause meningitis. Because the baby does not have the ability to fight infection the way an adult would, the infection can spread very rapidly and cause secondary effects that will not respond to antibiotics, like low blood pressure, low urine output, heart failure, and sepsis.

When a baby is admitted to the ICU nursery, infection is always considered. Screening tests are often obtained, and a decision by the medical team to place the baby on antibiotics will take into account lab work, a physical exam, and the medical history for the mother as well as the baby. It is very important for the mother to share all medical history from during the pregnancy and before the pregnancy with the NICU medical team so that the baby is able to receive the best therapy possible for infection.

The usual tests to screen for infection in babies include samples of blood, urine, spinal fluid, and sometimes mucous/sputum from the lungs. In some viral infections, your medical team may ask for samples from eye drainage, the skin, nasal drainage, or the rectum in addition to other routine blood work. Samples from any of these locations are known as cultures. Most blood cultures will take forty-eight to seventy-two hours for preliminary results to be obtained and as long as five to seven days for final results. Additionally, viral cultures and fungal cultures may take even longer, from ten to fourteen days. Your health care providers will use the results of these tests as well as the physical exam to determine the length of therapy. Occasionally, in special scenarios, an infectious disease specialist may be consulted to help the medical team determine the official length of therapy.

The most common infections seen in newborns include blood infections, urinary tract infections, lung infections, eye infections, skin infections, and meningitis. The most common types of bacteria that are seen in newborns include group B strep, E. coli, listeria, yeast, staphylococcus, herpes, chlamydia, gonorrhea, and viral infections such as the flu or RSV, respiratory syncytial virus. Your medical history is very important to help the medical team determine which organisms to consider and which medications to select, as many infants are born infected. Many of these conditions can be treated successfully. All babies with significant infections during the neonatal period will require close outpatient follow-up per the pediatrician.

In the NICU, one of the best ways to decrease your baby's risk for infection after birth is to follow the infection guidelines for the NICU. This includes following a strict handwashing technique, avoiding visiting if you have a cold, cough, or fever, and limiting the number of visitors that your baby may be exposed to while in the NICU. Finally, providing breast milk for your baby is one of the best ways to decrease the risk for infection in the NICU, especially a type of severe stomach infection that preemies can develop. The provision of breast milk for at least six months has also been shown to be protective later on for infants, decreasing the risk for viral infections, ear infections, and gastrointestinal problems. Even if your baby is unable to breastfeed or take breast milk by bottle, your baby can receive breast milk via a feeding tube. In the NICU, breast milk is not considered just a food, it is considered a medicine, and many NICUs are able to provide donor breast milk if a mother is unable to pump or has an inadequate supply.

Hopefully, your baby will not experience a severe infection, but if he or she does, be sure to ask your medical team these key questions: What type of infection does my baby have? How long will my baby require treatment? Will my baby require any other tests for this infection? Are you concerned about any long-term effects? Should I be worried about this infection in my other children? Please remember that most infections in neonates can be treated, but that each baby must be evaluated on an individual basis. Work with your medical team so that you are clear on the plan as well as the next steps. This will really help you to manage your anxiety and to continue to support your baby while in the NICU.

Questions for My Baby's Doctor

Notes about My Baby

CHAPTER 5

The Power of Breast Milk

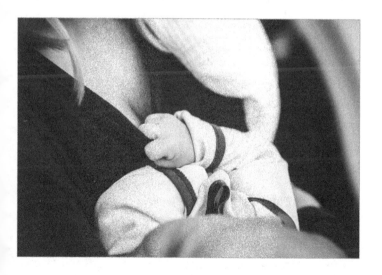

So, you've made it from the delivery room to admission to the NICU! You've made it through the scary breathing and respiratory talks. You've made it through the equally scary infection talks, and you are used to all the NICU alarms, monitors, beeps, and equipment! Now comes the fun part, eating, right? I always smile at this part because it seems so many parents are surprised at the actual steps that are involved with learning to suck, swallow, and breathe without choking. This is particularly true for parents who have a bigger preemie, one who is four or five pounds and at thirty-four or thirty-five weeks, because everyone knows someone who had a thirty-five-week preemie that went home with no problems. There is one thing I want to emphasize as a caveat to all parents of preemies and of term babies: if, for whatever reason, your baby needed to be admitted to the NICU for treatment or management, you cannot judge their progress based on other infants you see or hear about, as each course of treatment is going to be different. Try not to compare your baby to other preemies. I know it's hard, but you can do it!

So what about food? Glorious food. Most preemies and term infants will have feeds started as soon as the baby is stable with respect to respiratory and cardiac status. For most babies, this will occur between twelve and twenty-four hours. If not, it will occur as soon as your medical team deems the baby is stable enough to have food digested in the stomach. Several things can affect this determination: Is the baby awake? Does the baby have a normal oxygen and a normal blood pressure level? Is the baby having bowel movements? And, often most importantly, do we have breast milk? We know that most babies will tolerate breast milk better than formula and, as shared earlier, babies who receive breast milk in the NICU tend to have better outcomes and less risk for serious stomach infections.

Initially the baby will receive breast milk through a feeding tube if he or she is too immature to nipple or breathing too fast to take a bottle. Once the baby is older and more stable, the baby will be assessed by the bedside neonatal nurse and the occupational therapist to evaluate him or her for readiness to nipple. Babies are born knowing how to suck; this is a primitive reflex, and even twenty-two- and twenty-three-week-old babies can be seen prenatally on ultrasound sucking their thumbs. But can the baby suck, swallow, and breathe without choking? Many babies do not acquire this skill until thirty-six to thirty-eight weeks. Most NICU units will allow babies to start "practicing" or nuzzling at the breast at thirty-two to thirty-four weeks, depending on their maturing and their respiratory status. In this scenario, the mom will pump first and then the baby will practice nippling to avoid the baby getting too much milk and choking or, worse, aspirating. Aspirating is what happens when the milk accidently goes into the lungs, or "down the wrong pipe." Sometimes the baby's mouth may be too small to effectively nipple, so a nipple shield may be used; this allows the infant to suckle on the nipple shield while receiving milk into his or her tummy through a feeding tube.

Eventually, the baby will be strong enough to take some milk from the breast and have the remainder of what they need given by gavage tube or bottle. Nursing and occupational therapy will help the physician or practitioner determine how fast to advance the nipple feeds based on the baby's own effort. This is also known as cue-based feedings. Most babies are able to complete nippling safely between thirty-six to thirty-eight weeks, but some babies require longer, from thirty-eight to forty-two weeks. Each case must be evaluated on an individual basis to determine if there are other factors affecting the baby's ability to nipple well. Some of these factors include breathing problems, neurological problems, feeding aversion with possible reflux, and immaturity. Of note, most babies will be able to nipple or breastfeed just fine, but they need time… remember that, Mommy and Daddy, as time is the hardest part!

Questions for My Baby's Doctor

Notes about My Baby

CHAPTER 6

Preemies and Apnea of Prematurity

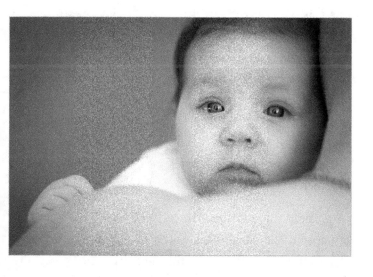

In addition to figuring out how to eat and continuing to gain weight, another thing your baby will have to accomplish before being able to be discharged home is continuing to breathe without apnea or a low heart rate. This is one of the main reasons that babies who are admitted to the intensive care nursery will remain on cardiac apnea monitors until they are discharged home. The part of the brain that reminds babies to breathe is not well developed until after thirty-five to thirty-seven weeks. Babies who are born at less than thirty-five weeks are routinely admitted to the NICU to have their breathing continuously monitored. The more immature a baby is, the more likely he or she is to have apnea. Apnea is defined as a period where the baby is not breathing, i.e. no chest movement, for twenty seconds. The longer the baby does not breathe, the more likely it is that the baby's heart rate will begin to drop. For babies at less than thirty weeks this is extremely common, and many will be routinely put on caffeine to help stimulate breathing. The caffeine is generally stopped around thirty-two to thirty-four weeks, and babies are monitored for ten to fourteen days off caffeine prior to discharge home.

When the monitor sounds that the baby is not breathing, the nurse will watch to see if this is a true alarm. If it is a true alarm and the baby is not breathing, the nurse will watch to see if the baby can self-recover; if the baby does not self-recover, the nurse will often stimulate the baby by rubbing the baby's back. If this does not work, the baby may require oxygen or support for breathing with a mask. The more episodes a baby has and the more severe individual episodes are, the more concerned the medical team will be that this is not just prematurity, but instead may be another concern, such as infection, feeding problems, seizures, or a brain problem. When a baby does have apnea, even if the baby is getting closer to discharge, the baby's discharge home must be delayed until the medical team is confident that the infant's breathing is more mature. This usually includes an additional monitoring period of five to seven days each time the baby has an episode of apnea. When it comes to shorthand, the interruption of breathing that is apnea is also referred to by the medical team as an *A*. The low heartrate that is bradycardia is also referred to by the medical team as a *B*. When the nurses are reporting on your infant to the medical team, they will often share how many As and Bs the baby had overnight. If your baby is on caffeine or has As and Bs, this is a question you should ask about when you are calling to check on your baby. This is particularly important as the baby gets closer to discharge, because it will affect how soon the baby is able to go home.

Questions for My Baby's Doctor

_____

_____

_____

_____

_____

_____

_____

Notes about My Baby

_____

_____

_____

_____

_____

_____

_____

CHAPTER 7

Will My Baby Be Normal?

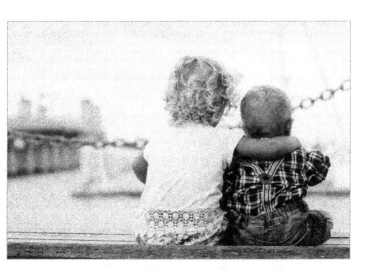

As I shared earlier in this book, this is the second most common question! Right after "Will my baby live?" we almost always hear "Will my baby be normal?" I hate this question and love this question. I hate this question because no one can predict the future, and statistics don't really matter to you if your baby is the one statistic that did not do well. But I also love this question because it means that the parents are thinking beyond the NICU. It means that you, Mom and Dad, are visualizing your baby in your home, as part of your family, and that is so important to maintain hope on the NICU journey.

Survival in the NICU improves after the first week in the NICU, particularly for the smallest and earliest of infants for whom those first several days are so critical. But so much of the outcome with respect to the remaining time in the NICU will depend on any complications that are associated with your child's course. A baby that has sicker lungs, needs more oxygen, or spends more time on the respirator will have a more complicated course. A baby who develops a severe infection which is complicated by meningitis or pneumonia will have a more complicated course. A baby who develops a problem in the NICU requiring surgery will have a more complicated course. A term baby who requires admission to the NICU for whatever reason will have a more complicated course. But what does it mean to have a more complicated course?

To have a complicated course just means that your baby may take longer to recover. That your baby may require more support and assistance after discharge. This does not mean that your baby does not have the potential to make a full recovery, but it does mean that you will have to pace yourself. Babies have a huge capacity to adapt and respond to therapy. I often see babies in the neonatal follow-up clinic who are doing much better than I anticipated. They may have taken longer to eat and required a feeding tube to go home; they may have taken longer to walk and required additional surgery or support; they may have required eye surgery but have adequate vision with glasses; but these are conditions that babies have the capacity to adapt to with time. Will they have the course they may have had, had they never been premature or never sick or never required surgery? It is unlikely, but no one really knows the answer to that… but what we do know is that most babies can and will improve with time.

One thing for parents to remember with premature babies is that they will develop based on their true gestational age… not their birth date. So, if a baby is born at thirty weeks and a normal pregnancy is forty weeks, that baby is ten weeks or two and a half months early. This means that when the baby is twelve months chronological age, the baby will be nine and a half months corrected age. Most babies will walk between ten and fifteen months of age, with the average being twelve months. A thirty-week preemie, though twelve months of age, will likely walk closer to fourteen to fifteen months of age, because that is when he or she would be twelve months for corrected age. Premature babies will follow their gestational age, and a pediatrician that works with preemies will generally follow their corrected age until age three.

So what is normal? Is normal being able to run, to walk, to play? Is normal being able to read, to write, to draw, to sing? Is normal the capacity to know and give love? You will have to determine that for your family. When the medical team is speaking to families about "normal," we are sharing statistics that define normal as being without major handicap. "Without major handicap" is defined as, for example, not having cerebral palsy, not being blind, or not having a lung disease that required a tracheostomy. There are many, many levels in between, and lots of gray areas, Mom and Dad.

The smallest and sickest babies will be at risk to have the most severe medical and neurological outcomes. This includes bleeding in the brain that could lead to cerebral palsy, eye disease that could lead to blindness, and lung disease that could lead to a tracheostomy. There are several levels of severity for bleeding in the brain, scar tissue to the eyes, and scar tissue to the lungs, all of which will have to be followed long-term to determine the ultimate outcome. We are able to provide very general information in the NICU… but the true course will be determined as your son or daughter is followed developmentally through the first three years of life. If there are concerns due to complications that your child is at risk for developmental delay or neurological compromise, be sure to speak with your medical team about options for therapy and follow-up once your infant is discharged, as well as options for supportive care at home if your infant is incapacitated or expected to have a shorter than normal life span. Continue to ask questions and reach out to other families who have cared for babies who have similar conditions to your baby. I have found that other families are the best allies for supporting your family.

Questions for My Baby's Doctor

_____

_____

_____

_____

_____

_____

_____

Notes about My Baby

_____

_____

_____

_____

_____

_____

CHAPTER 8

What About Preemie Surgeries?

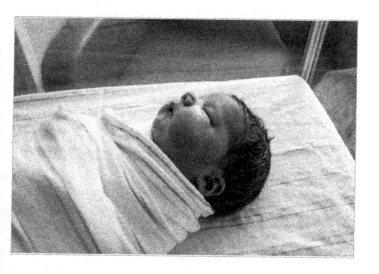

So, this chapter might be a tad bit scary. Most babies who are admitted to the NICU nursery will not require surgery. Many will merely require continuous monitoring once their breathing and heart rate are stabilized. Once they are big enough, old enough, and stable enough, they will begin to work on feeding and will, hopefully, eventually be able to go home. But this is still an intensive care nursery and not a regular nursery, and, unfortunately, sometimes babies will become very sick, often critically ill. These critically ill babies may require lifesaving measures, including surgery. Some of these conditions may respond to antibiotics, respiratory support, or intravenous fluids, but other conditions may only respond to surgery, and even then the baby may remain critically ill and ultimately may not survive.

There are many conditions that a baby may require surgery for in the intensive care nursery; fortunately, most of these conditions are rare… but some conditions, particularly for premature infants, are more frequent. If your baby is diagnosed with a condition that will require surgery, you will be updated initially by the medical team in the NICU and then later by the pediatric surgeon who will be performing your baby's surgery.

The purpose of this chapter is just to provide a general overview of some of the more common conditions that may require surgery in the neonatal period. More extensive information will be provided by your medical team.

In preemies, the most common types of surgery include heart surgery, eye surgery, brain surgery, and stomach surgery. With respect to heart surgery, the most common reason for it in a preemie is a surgery to clip or close a vessel called a PDA (patent ductus arteriosus). The PDA is a special blood vessel that is between the heart and the lungs. It is a blood vessel that all babies have that normally closes on its own in the first several days of life. This blood vessel serves a purpose when the baby is still in the womb, but once the baby is born its presence can lead the baby to have heart failure. It can be treated with medicine initially, but if it continues to cause problems, especially for preemies, your doctor may recommend surgery.

The need for eye surgery can be one of the most serious complications of prematurity. The more premature an infant is, the more at risk the infant may be for scar tissue to the eyes because of prematurity and high levels of oxygen exposure. Although the medical team may work very hard to minimize the need for extra oxygen exposure for your infant, often, if the lungs are very premature, especially for twenty-two- to twenty-five-week infants, they may still need high levels of oxygen to survive. However, high levels of oxygen exposure can cause the blood vessels in the eyes of very premature infants, those less than thirty-two weeks, to develop abnormally. This abnormal development is called ROP, or retinopathy of prematurity. If there is enough scar tissue, the blood vessels can pull on the retina and the retina may detach. Premature infants who are born at less than thirty-two weeks will have their first eye exam at four to six weeks of age, depending on the infant's gestational age. After the initial exam, the infant will be routinely evaluated by the pediatric ophthalmologist every two to four weeks until they are discharged to evaluate for ROP and the need for possible surgery.

One of the most serious complications of premature babies is a life-threatening stomach infection known as NEC, or necrotizing enterocolitis. It is particularly scary because it usually does not show up until two to three weeks of age, and usually in a preterm infant that is currently stable. NEC involves a severe stomach infection whereby the bacteria causes the intestines to be very inflamed, leading to bloody stools and sometimes an actual hole in the intestine, which requires emergency surgery. Some babies can be treated with antibiotics, as well as by allowing the bowels to rest by not feeding the baby for a week or more. Other babies will require surgery to remove the dead bowel tissue and, sometimes, to set up the placement of a colostomy or ileostomy.

This infection can be very severe, and babies can lose a large amount of their intestinal tract. This can unfortunately lead to lifelong problems with digestion and growth. Of note, babies can also develop a spontaneous hole in the intestines in the first week of life, even before feeding, which also requires surgery and can lead to complications later with respect to feeding, growth, and nutrition. Often, in both NEC and spontaneous perforation, infants will require a longer period on IV nutrition, which can lead to other complications, particularly with respect to the liver. Physicians, practitioners, and nurses are very vigilant about monitoring for this infection in your infant. This is the reason why feeds are advanced cautiously, stool is documented, and the stomach is evaluated for digestion of contents before each feed. If there are any concerns, feeding can be interrupted and the infant screened before resuming. If your baby develops a stomach infection, be sure to ask the medical team if they believe your baby will require surgery to manage the infection. One of the ways to prevent this complication is for the baby to receive breast milk instead of formula.

Some premature babies will develop a major complication as a result of stress, low blood pressure, and immaturity, which will lead to bleeding in the brain. If the bleeding in the brain is significant enough, the baby may develop swelling of the brain, known as hydrocephalus. In a premature infant with possible hydrocephalus, it is important to monitor the physical exam for signs of increased cranial pressure. This includes clinical signs such as seizures, lethargy, or vomiting, or if the brain is not growing. If your baby shows these signs, your medical team will likely consult the pediatric neurosurgeon. The pediatric neurosurgeon may recommend additional tests such as a CT or MRI to better evaluate how the brain is growing with the hydrocephalus and to determine if the baby needs the fluid to be drained. If the pediatric neurosurgeon decides that the fluid needs to be drained, he can place special tubing into one of the channels or ventricles of the brain which will allow the excess fluid to be drained out of the brain via shunt, usually into the abdomen. He can also place a reservoir in the brain if the infant is too small for a shunt, which will allow the medical team to remove fluid from the reservoir as needed.

In addition to the most common surgical problems of premature infants, many term infants will also require admission to the intensive care nursery for surgery for birth defects. Sometimes these problems have been diagnosed prior to birth, but many times they may not be realized until after the baby is born. The list of these types of problems is long. Some of the more common surgical procedures for birth defects include: heart surgery for missing parts or abnormal functioning of the heart; stomach surgery if part of the intestine did not develop normally, if part of the intestine is blocked, if part of the intestine is found in the chest or outside of the body, or if part of the GI tract, like the anus, is missing; spinal cord surgery if part of the spinal cord is open; surgery for a cleft lip or cleft palate if the mouth and nose did not form normally; esophageal surgery if the esophagus did not form normally; nares surgery if the nose is blocked; eye surgery if an infant is born with hemorrhages, cataracts, or glaucoma; and support for positional deformities if the bones are abnormal in the feet or hands or if the clavicle is broken.

Although these conditions sound very serious, the initial stabilization—as mentioned in Chapter 4—always revolves around breathing and stabilization of the heart. Following the stabilization of those two organ systems, the specialist for your baby's specific condition will be consulted on the best course of action for your baby. If your baby does require surgery, you will likely be meeting many people. Be sure to keep a notepad handy to record all the names of the individuals you may meet, the information that is shared, and any questions you may have regarding your baby's plan of care.

Questions for My Baby's Doctor

Notes about My Baby

CHAPTER 9

. . . .

Caring for Your Baby in the NICU

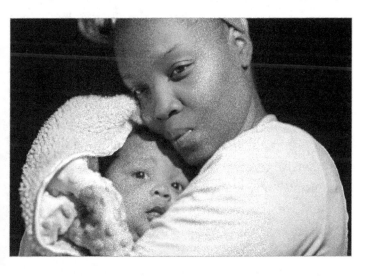

Although this chapter is at the end of the book, step nine in your path to navigating the NICU journey for your Early Arrival, it's perhaps the most important step...

and maybe should be Chapter 1! When a parent has a baby admitted to the NICU, the initial response is, understandably, shock. How did this happen? Is this really happening? Is my baby going to be okay? Will my baby go home with me? And then, when Mom and Dad are finally able to visit their baby in the ICU nursery (which may be hours later if the baby required stabilization) they are greeting with alarms, beepers, noises, and rules in a world most people have not visited… and many would prefer never to visit again. So how do parents begin to make sense of the chaos that is the NICU? How does one manage being an advocate for their baby? Constantly being asked questions about consenting for care, but still being in a fog about what said care actually entails, because the baby is not supposed to be here yet! Or, if the baby is supposed to be here, a term baby, the baby is supposed to be here in your room, with you… not in the intensive care nursery connected to wires, monitors, and intravenous lines. It's such a tough transition for families, whether the baby is big or whether the baby is small… no one wants to be in the intensive care nursery. This is quite humbling for me as an intensive care nursery physician. Every day I will meet someone who did not want to meet me. Who was not planning to meet me, and who, presumably, I will have to share news with that is at the least very upsetting and at the most devastating. How does one navigate that void?

So, how does one move as a parent from questioning to acceptance? How do you move from asking: What is wrong with my baby? Will my baby be okay? Will my baby survive? And instead start saying: Yes, my baby is sick. Yes, this is not what I had planned. Yes, I am sad. But I am still Mommy. I am still Daddy… and I want my baby to know that I am here. I want to know that my baby will be okay, at least for today… I need to know that. I will worry about tomorrow when tomorrow comes. It sounds like such a simple approach, but in practice it takes a while to accept the parts of this journey that, unfortunately, we can't change… and to look at the parts of the journey that will enable and encourage you as a parent.

One of the ways to do this is to make sure, when you visit, to touch your baby. It may seem scary at first. The baby may be really tiny. The baby may be struggling to breathe. But your baby knows you. Your nurses will be able to show you how to gently place your thumb in your baby's palm so that your baby can grab your finger. Speak softly. Your baby knows your voice. He or she has already heard it through the womb. Call their name. Name your baby. Sometimes families are afraid to name their babies because they are afraid the baby is too sick and they are afraid of becoming attached. But your baby is here now, today, in this moment… this minute… this hour… and they need a name. Trust your gut to give them a name and then speak it and cherish it. Once your baby is more stable, and especially once your baby no longer has any intravenous lines in the umbilical cord, be sure to ask the medical team when you can hold your baby. Even very tiny babies can be held skin to skin on the chest. This is called kangaroo care and is great for bonding, for both Mom and Dad and especially for the baby. Once the baby is on your chest, consider reading to the baby, sharing your favorite scriptures, singing to the baby, or just watching the baby through a hand mirror. You will find that kangaroo care will become a very special time for both you and your baby.

Another way to promote your bonding in the NICU is to begin to journal when you come to visit your baby. It doesn't have to be long, just a few words: Today I watched you ____. Today I am feeling ____. Today you had a rough day. Today you had a good day. Tomorrow we are looking forward to ____. You will be amazed at the progress both you and your child will make over the NICU stay.

For those of you with very premature infants, be sure to document firsts. When infants are in the NICU for two, three, four, even five months, it can be very hard to see the light at the end of the tunnel, so you have to light the candles... find your way. Document the firsts. NICU parents have an appreciation for firsts that parents of well infants may not have and often take for granted. When did you first hear your baby cry? If your baby was very sick, you may not have heard that in the delivery room. When did you first get to hold your baby? Most parents of preemies can tell you the first day they finally got to hold their baby. When did your baby first have all IVs removed? When did your baby have his or her first breastfeed or bottle? When did your baby first become big enough to get out of the isolette?

The first day where you have to go home and your baby stays in the hospital will be tough. You come into the hospital pregnant, but you leave the hospital not pregnant and without your baby. You may go home to an empty nursery or you may no longer be looking forward to your baby shower. These are normal emotions; be sure to talk to your spouse or significant other or to a close friend about them, as well as to your NICU social worker, bedside nurse, or medical team. We are here to support you through this transition. You are part of the medical team, and our first job is to support your role as parent and to facilitate bonding, in addition to making sure you are informed with respect to medical decision making. You can do this, Mom and Dad... but pace yourself. One day at a time. And we will be here to help you navigate the way.

It's tough having a baby in the NICU... but you are here now. Let us know how we can help you. Start from the beginning and work your way to the end, and please remember that you are not alone.

Nine steps! You can do this. Breathe. Welcome to the NICU!

1. Identify the medical team.

2. Identify the equipment.

3. Remember, breathing is our focus in the beginning.

4. Watch out for infection.

5. Commit to breastfeeding.

6. Apnea is real... it takes time to mature.

7. Normal is relative... the best is yet to come.

8. Watch for serious complications... and ask questions.

9. But most of all, don't forget to be Mom and Dad! It's time to bond!

Questions for My Baby's Doctor

Notes about My Baby

THANK YOU

I am not sure what led you to get *Early Arrival: 9 Things Parents Need to Know about Life in the ICU Nursery: A Doctor's Step-by-Step Guide*, but I am glad that you did. If you currently have a baby in the ICU nursery or you are supporting someone who has a baby in the ICU nursery... my prayers are with you. The NICU journey is filled with uncertainty, anxiety, and chaos! This leads to some really incredible highs and some equally devastating lows, but most families will navigate the journey and be stronger for the experience. I wish that no babies were ever born sick. I wish that no parent ever had to enter the NICU. But, for those of you who do, I hope that this book gives you just a little hope, a little light, and a little confidence for your journey. You can do this. Please keep in touch and let me know how your little one is doing. Let me know what you would like to see in the next edition of this book. Let me know the parts you liked the best and the parts you liked the least. It is my hope and prayer that this book will be a true asset for NICU families, and I will continue to work to make sure that it meets your expectations. Wishing you love, light, and laughter for the journey! Let's keep in touch!

WEBSITE:
www.drterrimd.com

FACEBOOK:
https://www.facebook.com/DrTerriMD

TWITTER:
https://twitter.com/drterrimd

YOUTUBE:
https://www.youtube.com/channel/UCm9s27Y-8ga-QQdSJXeb-oGw?disable_polymer=true

INSTAGRAM:
https://www.instagram.com/doctorterrimd/

LINKED IN:
https://www.linkedin.com/in/drterrimd/

POSTSCRIPT: WHEN HELLO MEANS GOODBYE

I've been blessed to care for babies and families for over twenty years. In that capacity, I am able to see a miracle every single day... there's nothing quite like being able to hold a tiny human in your hand, watching that baby grow big and strong against all odds and one day be able to go home with his or her parents. Fortunately, that's the case for most of my patients... but, sadly, not all of them. While I look forward to the day when no parent has to say goodbye to their baby, I know that that day is not yet here, so this chapter is for the angel babies... those miracle babies to whom parents have to say both hello and goodbye.

First, let me begin by saying I am so sorry for your loss. I don't know your story... but I do know the pain of having to tell a parent that their baby is not going to survive. There is really no way to say those words without sadness, without pain, so I will not try to do that here.

But what I would like to say is that, if you find yourself on the receiving end of those words and you have time, have a moment to gather your thoughts, you should take that moment, if you are able, to share with your medical team how you would like to honor the life of your child. In what way would you like to create a memory with your child during the sacred time you have to say good-bye... the special time you have with your baby while they are here?

If your medical team has not asked you about your wishes, but has delivered news that suggests that your baby may not survive, you can ask them. Even at a time where it seems you have no choices... you do still have some choices, sweet friend, and one of those choices is how you choose to say hello and goodbye to your precious little one.

One way that parents' can still have choices at this most difficult time is through neonatal palliative care or perinatal hospice. Many families, when initially approached about perinatal hospice or neonatal palliative care for a critically ill infant, may initially refuse as the idea is understandably frightening and brings with it a natural degree of sadness. However, once you have a moment to process, to grieve, you may be able to find some comfort in the opportunity to have some control in how you want to say good-bye to your infant—at a time when it seems like you may not have had control over so many other circumstances. This includes time of delivery, time of labor, presence of birth defects, and unfortunate events that happen to a baby that was once very stable. Whatever the cause, it's all heartbreaking, and those feelings will continue to bring sadness.

One way to deal with the sadness for many families is neonatal palliative care and even perinatal hospice. Palliative care, in its simplest form, is care that improves the quality of life for a patient. Many families associate palliative care automatically with hospice care, but hospice care is only one part of palliative care. Palliative care includes systems and process of providing care, physical care, emotional support, spiritual support, cultural support, pain control, end of life care and ethical issues related to the care of patients with life-limiting illnesses. For babies receiving neonatal palliative care, all of these domains are really important to supporting families from the moment of diagnosis.

Perinatal hospice is actually a very unique branch of palliative and hospice medicine that has only fully emerged in the past 15 years as a very important means to care for families of infants with lethal birth defects. Perinatal hospice may be offered to families for whom the parents have received a prenatal diagnosis that suggests that the infant may not survive the pregnancy or survive an extended period after delivery. In those instances, a plan is carefully created to maximize the time that the family will have with the child at delivery, often including baptism and photography at delivery, as this may be the only time the family has with their child. Additionally, families are encouraged to create moments during the pregnancy as part of their parenting journey, as for many, this sadly will be the majority of their parenting experience.

Whatever the circumstances surrounding your baby and your baby's illness, please know that you do have choices. Even in the direst of circumstances, you still have choices. Sometimes the choice may just be to hold your baby for as long as you want; sometimes it may be to see your baby again even after someone has taken him or her away. Your Neonatal and Labor and Delivery team will be able to support you. Please don't hesitate to ask for what you need. I'll be sending hugs and prayers for peace and strength your way!

Some questions that may help you to create a plan during this difficult time include:

1. Do you want to have the baby baptized?

2. Do you want to take pictures with the baby?

3. Do you want the baby to receive some support, such as oxygen or pain medication, if it would be deemed helpful by the medical team?

4. Do you want the baby to receive some breast milk or colostrum as a comfort measure if able?

5. Would you like to bathe the baby?

6. Do you want to try to take the baby home if possible? If so, would you like to explore options for pediatric hospice?

7. Do you have a special outfit you would like the baby to wear?

8. Are there siblings we need to support?

9. Which family members would you like to have present during your time with the baby?

10. Are there special ceremonies or rituals that you would like the baby to participate in during the time you are saying goodbye?

11. Would you like the baby to remain in the room with you?

Dear Mom and Dad... If you are reading this chapter... I imagine it means that you have had to say goodbye to your sweet baby too soon. Although this is a part of my job, it never gets easier... and I look forward to the day when no one has to say goodbye to their baby. I hope that, in the moments... hours... days that you were able to spend with your little one, your medical team showed you compassion. That you got to hold your baby. That you know that your baby knew you and experienced love. May your angel baby rest in peace and may you continue to speak his or her name... and please know... you are not alone.

DR. TERRIS TOP 5 QUESTIONS FOR THE NICU MEDICAL TEAM

1. **What are you most concerned about today for my baby?** It seems like such a simple and obvious question, but parents and physicians are often concerned about two very different things. Parents have often heard lots of scary numbers prior to the delivery of their baby... and they continue to wonder: is my baby going to live? It's helpful to ask those questions. Similarly, sometimes the medical team, in an effort to protect the family, may not always clearly demonstrate to the family what the main concern is for the baby today, in this moment, and that information can be invaluable for families.

2. **What medications are being given to my baby and why?** When premature babies are born, it's often a life-threatening emergency. Many forms are signed. Many conditions explained. It can be a blur. But once the dust settles, if the dust settles, the treatment plan

often changes. You may know what medicines your baby is receiving, but what are the side effects of those medications? How long does the medical team expect the baby to be on those medications?

3. **When can I hold my baby?** Often, and unfortunately, premature babies are too sick, too small, and have too much needed equipment to be held. Initially this is understandable, as the main purpose of the medical team is the medical care of the infant. However, I do believe that, more often than not, babies can be held—and often babies do fine… sometimes better than expected. I also think that, at times, the power of human touch, the power of parents to bond with their infant, can really help, as well as be a rite of parenthood. We sometimes forget, as the days turn into weeks and the weeks turn into months, that a mother or father has not been able to hold their child. Each case must be weighed carefully, but ask… and ask again. The answer may be *no* today, but it may be *yes* tomorrow. These moments are priceless… and therapeutic for both baby and parents. It can be frightening to hold a one pound baby; but, parents, you can do it, and your NICU staff will help you.

4. **If this treatment does not work, what are our other options?** Premature babies can become very sick

very quickly. The field has grown tremendously; even in the last five years we are saving babies that we would not have been able to save ten years ago. We are doing surgeries while infants are still in the womb. We are helping infants to start breastfeeding earlier. Parents are sometimes able to live in the NICU. We are putting fewer babies on the respirator. This is all very exciting, but even our best equipment, our best medicines, will at times fall short. If your baby is sick or becomes very unstable after having been stable, ask your physician or practitioner if there are other options. Often, other options are not initially shared because they may be too risky or they may be too overwhelming for parents; because of this, parents may believe we have already offered everything possible when we may be able to offer more, or they may believe we can offer more when in fact we have offered all we can. These are difficult conversations... but they are the basis for informed decision making, and necessary for parents to be the best advocates they can be for their child.

5. **Do you anticipate any long-term complications from this illness?** Being able to survive the NICU is only a part of the battle. Many premature babies will go on to experience problems with lung disease,

requiring oxygen; problems with vision, including blindness; problems with growth; problems with feeding; and problems with overall developmental delay... even big preemies can have these issues. Fortunately, there are many services in place to assist families with navigating the journey after leaving the neonatal intensive care unit. It is important to be aware of possible long-term complications so that, in the event these problems arise, a plan can be in place to make sure your child can get the care they need so they can achieve their greatest potential.

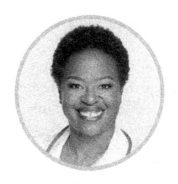

ABOUT THE AUTHOR

Dr. Terri Major-Kincade is a board-certified pediatrician and neonatologist and a pioneer in the field of neonatal palliative care. She has been featured on ABC's Houston Medical and Lifetime's Women Docs and is frequently a keynote speaker at national pediatric, obstetric, and palliative care conferences. Her mission is to empower families to make informed choices for their babies at a time when they believe they have no choice, as well as to empower physicians and nurses to help families making those difficult choices. She strongly believes that, while it is not possible to save every baby, finding hope in the midst of despair is a gift that benefits both families and staff as they do their very best to care for both the family and the baby.

In addition to supporting families directly in the NICU, Dr. Major-Kincade has been an avid volunteer with the March of Dimes, leading several initiatives to bring awareness to the crisis of preterm birth and health disparities with respect to poor birth outcomes, and she has an interest in long-term follow-up of NICU graduates.

Dr. Terri lives in Dallas, Texas, with her husband and two children.

CREATING DISTINCTIVE BOOKS
WITH INTENTIONAL RESULTS

We're a collaborative group of creative masterminds with a mission to produce high-quality books to position you for monumental success in the marketplace.

Our professional team of writers, editors, designers, and marketing strategists work closely together to ensure that every detail of your book is a clear representation of the message in your writing.

Want to know more?
Write to us at info@publishyourgift.com
or call (888) 949-6228

Discover great books, exclusive offers, and more at
www.PublishYourGift.com

Connect with us on social media

@publishyourgift

CPSIA information can be obtained
at www.ICGtesting.com
Printed in the USA
FSHW04n1334190418
47003FS